GUIDED MEDITATION FOR DEEP SLEEP, RELAXATION AND STRESS RELIEF

RELAX YOUR BODY AND MIND, OVERCOME DEPRESSION, ANXIETY AND INSOMNIA WITH RELAXATION TECHNIQUES

The information in the following pages is broadly considered a truthful and accurate account of facts and as such, any inattention, use, or misuse of the information in question by the reader will render any resulting actions solely under their purview. There are no scenarios in which the publisher or the original author of this work can be in any fashion deemed liable for any hardship or damages that may befall them after undertaking information described herein.

Additionally, the information in the following pages is intended only for informational purposes and should thus be thought of as universal. As befitting its nature, it is presented without assurance regarding its prolonged validity or interim quality. Trademarks that are mentioned are done without written consent and can in no way be considered an endorsement from the trademark holder.

TABLE OF CONTENT

INTRODUCTION

Guided meditation simply uses meditation help and is the perfect way to introduce a person to the world of meditation.

This is the new relaxing technique for the busy lives of today and is also good for beginners who find meditation difficult to concentrate. Most people practice guided meditation to relieve their daily stress and to create a style of life full of happiness, good health, and plenty.

When you practice meditation from an experienced mentor, there will be harmony, serenity and calm. Eventually, with regular training you will open up new ideas.

You can use meditation to ground and concentrate or offer healing power to relieve everything you need. You should ask for advanced therapy, such as Dynamic Meditation, from your higher intelligence.

You can be inspired, open to grace and empathy, refresh your physical equipment or just remember your true depth.

Guided meditation can help you concentrate on yourself to bring inner peace and relaxation, or focus on your relationship with God or your spiritual life. Anyway, after meditation you will find yourself in a more peaceful, peaceful and restful place.

This can include body relaxation and wonderful spiritual growth. Relaxation Meditation Relaxation methods can help you feel calmer and more in keeping with your daily tasks. It has shown that a meditative relaxing state accompanies and causes a person to feel less depressed and controlled all day long.

A person who is experienced in meditation can do his own research and exploration in meditation. There are a variety of positive health effects, stress management and cure, such as great relaxation, improved sleep patterns and strengthening of the immune system.

While meditation is not clinically shown to heal people of physical problems, it is a good way for people to concentrate and think about their physical health. Many have witnessed miraculous healing signs without any medical explanation.

It is also understood that meditation makes a person not only more relaxed but also more focused and troublesome. Meditation can, through a guide, not just become a healthy way to deal with tension, but also a good way for people to better themselves and fix their personal problems.

There don't seem to be many good choices when talking about how and where you will find plenty in your life right now. You need to make your feelings, your aura, your being and your environment multiply.

This is the nature of the Law of Attraction, which can be used for meditation. Whether you want more wealth and riches or abundance in all areas of your life, meditation is the best place to begin the process, particularly dynamic meditation. It helps you to enjoy your life and to earn plenty.

Directed meditation is a very common way to get started because it needs a professional teacher who guides you by a directed approach that helps you sense the beauty, peace and love meditation. During this wonderful journey, inner peace is generated and your meaning in life will be known, if you wish.

It is the best way to meditate and the best way. It is also one of the simplest and most informative ways to control your life in every way. Most of them seek a deeper understanding of their own spiritual reality and want to continue on a clear journey from ancient times. Guided mediation sets you on the road to the direction of your destiny.

CHAPTER 1

What Is Guided Meditation?

Guided meditation (sometimes called guided visual meditation) is just "guided meditation." This is one of the best ways to enter a state of deep relaxation and internal peace, and is one of the most effective ways to remove tension and make positive personal changes.

How is this?

Guided meditations are usually performed using a meditation teacher or listening to a recording.

You can sit comfortably, or you may be asked to lie down in some situations. Then you listen to your guide as they lead you through a number of relaxing visualizations. When you slowly relax and become calm, tension decreases, and the mind becomes clearer and clearer.

Whilst you are in this deeply comfortable state of mind, your subconscious is open to constructive advice, and this time your guide will take you on a path that enhances one or more aspects of your life. For instance, a guided meditation can be adapted to personal empowerment and positive thinking.

Another could concentrate on emotional cure or spiritual development. You could take a guided journey to unleash all your potential, or simply go on a guided journey for the sheer joy of deep relaxation.

As you can see now, guided meditation can be not only relaxing, but also enhancing your feeling for yourself, transforming your perspective in a positive way and inspiring you to live your lives to the full.

It is a smooth, pleasant experience which leads to deep relaxation, stress elimination and an enhanced appreciation of life.

At the end of your meditation, your guide will take you back to normal consciousness, leaving you refreshed, rejuvenated and relaxed.

A guided meditation may take as little as five minutes or an hour, depending on your personal preference. In most cases, a guided meditation of 20 minutes or longer is recommended if a real depth of relaxation is to be experienced and the positive benefits maximized.

Who distinguishes guided meditation?

Many conventional meditation techniques allow you to take control of your own consciousness by focusing your attention on a single focal point. This focus can be your breath, it may be a physical action, or more often it can be on a mantra-the sound, the word, or the phrase you mentally repeat.

While these effective methods of meditation are excellent to create inner relaxation and to improve the ability to focus, some people find it hard to regulate.

Among the main reasons why guided meditations are so popular as traditional meditation is because they do not require any prior training or effort.

Even if you are someone who find it extremely difficult to let go of some thoughts, even though you are overloaded with mental activity or highly stressed, when properly guided, you can quickly achieve peace and quiet.

Because this type of meditation is so easy, it is very helpful for new people. However, guided meditations can also be of great benefit to meditative experts.

Experienced meditators often use guided visualization meditation to undergo a more intense or vivid relaxation, to dig more deeply into their minds than they usually do or to discuss a specific aspect of personal development.

Guided meditation also differs from traditional meditation as it uses music and the sounds of nature to improve your experience of meditation.

The role of music and nature sounds in guided imaging meditation Guided imaging meditation recording usually includes soothing relaxation music, which helps you to relax while guided by meditation.

Think of how much a good soundtrack makes for a film. Guided meditations benefit similarly from music. Music adds to your guided journey of meditation another dimension of expression and depth while soothing your mind.

It is also not unusual for CDs and MP3s of guided meditation to include sounds of nature. These sounds are extremely relaxing, and can also be used in the meditation to enhance the vibrancy of visualizations.

For example, if you are directed to imagine yourself on a sandy beach, your visualization experience will be more realistic, if you really hear the sound of seawaves.

Unlike conventional meditation, which seeks to achieve cognitive relaxation through concentration exercises, guided imaging meditations use an imaginative tapestry of visualizations, music and ambient sounds to relax, captivate your mind, and immerse you in an inner journey.

Due to the fact that this inner voyage can be tailored to specific results, guided meditation can be even more powerful than traditionally passive techniques when it comes to positive personal changes in your life.

Guided Meditation is a taping usually made by professional people, such as yoga teachers, life coaches or hypnotherapists. All you need to do is listen to the recording (ideally through headphones) in a peaceful position where you will not be distracted and your body will do the rest for you.

A guided meditation lasts from 10 minutes to an hour and even 10 minutes will help calm you down and center you. The best recordings often combine a soothing voice with gentle relaxing music.

The recordings of the meditation usually follow the same format. The speaker first brings you to a place of profound relaxation, and then takes you to a profound meditative state. A place where your mind can rest and relax.

In many different situations a guided meditation can be used. Many Guided Meditations can now be accessed through Internet downloads. This allows you to listen to your MP3 or PC meditation and a CD player, so you can play them in a wide variety of settings and integrate them in your daily routines.

I have a variety of drugs that I use for different lengths in different situations stored on my iPlayer. I consider that a 15-minute mediation record is just perfect for a long journey or train break. The longer meditations I often do at home if I want to spend an hour or even at night before I go to sleep.

The only way that you can really feel the advantages of this meditation is to try it for yourself. Most shops have guided meditation CDs, but you don't have to purchase a whole CD to try one. Individual tracks of different lengths for less than $1 can be downloaded.

There are so many advantages of meditation. These include better sleep habits, more flexibility throughout the day, better working conditions and a less nervous or depressed feeling for a few.

Even after just one session, you will see an improvement in your stress levels, but since the advantages are cumulative, we advise you to try your Guided Meditation for a week every day and then you can really see the more relaxed you feel and the more comfortable your day-to-day lives are.

Meditation can be as old as mankind. Different techniques were used by similar meditators in different parts of the world at different times throughout the long history of meditation.

Several types of meditation exist today, but "guided meditation" is one of the most common. It is a technique of meditation best suited for beginners because no training or effort is needed beforehand.

Only experienced meditators may find it most helpful, however. A "guided meditation" means simply using some verbal instructions to slowly bring you into a state of consciousness.

In your meditative experience, you are driven by a voice-either live or recorded. A soothing voice can direct the imagination on a particular path in order to achieve some general or specific objective.

The aim is usually to calm the mind and achieve deep relaxation. Those with a particular purpose could include: recovery, self-improvement, removal of a negative programming, behavior change or release negative emotions that hinder you. Those meditations use the power of visualizations to bring about positive personal changes.

Some evoke higher states of consciousness and stimulate energies sleeping in human bodies.

Most guided meditation lasts just five minutes, some take 40 or more minutes. Many use quiet meditative music during the recording or live experience.

You are asked to sit or lie comfortably in order to start the relaxation sequence. You will be moved by a kind voice until you are deeply relaxed. It will remind you not to chat but to draw attention to your breath.

You will be asked to bring your focus into your body and relax deeply. Most guided meditations ask you to visualize pictures of some experiences and emotions.

The sub consciousness is open to constructive feedback once we enter the state of deep relaxation. This can be the focus of the guided meditation or you can only use it to relax and reduce stress.

You are progressively returned to a state of normal consciousness, feeling refreshed and relaxed.

Guided meditations can be done via blogs, mobile applications, podcasts and CDs in a class. You can have someone speak to you or read a guided meditation, or play it back to yourself. With this album, you can carry your meditative experiences wherever you go and use them at any time.

CHAPTER 2

Forms of Guided Meditation

In the fast-moving world in which we live today, stress and anxiety are inherent in our lives. If the people around you, your job or your present circumstances continually pressure you, relaxation can be just what you need to break free from these negative aspects.

This is a way to reduce stress and can make us experience inner peace, tranquility or even harmony with the supreme power and universe.

In addition, meditation is also for those who want to achieve success and breakthroughs in their lives or overcome obstacles in certain fields. There are never ending reasons why people meditate, but it is always to produce a positive result.

Two types of guided meditations are mostly accessible-individual guided meditation and group guided meditation.

Individual guided meditation-a meditation that is done by itself, usually in a comfortable environment to physically relax. A popular method is to use a MP3 or DVD audio therapy, in which calming music and subliminal messages direct a person through a visual and creative journey.

Group Guided Meditation is a group meditation led by a meditation instructor. It is a group meditation. Since the teacher is present physically to support or to provide immediate feedback, guided community meditation generally produces greater results than meditation alone.

It also provides a platform for participants to connect with other like-minded individuals where they can be motivated to gather new ideas or learn different meditation techniques.

Those are two broad types of meditation, whether performed in groups or individually: audiopedication—meditation is done by listening to an audio-guided path of meditation with vocal instructions to instill new beliefs and visualize the success or breakthroughs that are needed.

It is usually accompanied in the background by serene music. This helps you achieve mental and emotional balance, quietness and stability. Mindfulness meditation teaches practitioners to focus and focus on their current state of feelings, feelings, actions and even breath.

Through this, practitioners will have the opportunity to learn about their thoughts and raise awareness about their environment and current actions.

Practitioners also find that they will enjoy living fully in the moment instead of being mentally present in the past and the future. We start to love and accept themselves, without making themselves harsh judgments.

Yes, meditation gives us a lot of advantages. This alleviates our negative thoughts, improves health and helps us achieve the breakthroughs and achievement that we are after.

Perhaps importantly, it gives us the opportunity to better understand ourselves and find ways to create new systems to handle anxieties and pressure. You won't see a new and better YOU long before you!

Every form of meditation can benefit physiologically, emotionally and psychologically. Guided meditations focus your mind while still allowing you to escape the daily activity and constant talk. Using your imagination and guided meditation, you will naturally find peace and happiness by letting your mind peacefully.

This simple exercise depends on how you relax with your imagination. Read the directions first and then try for yourself. Picture yourself in a sunny place, comfortable and warm. It can be a spot you've been before or just imagined. See you sitting here feel very safe and safe. Feel bathed in the warmth of the warm sun. Take the sun, feel it bathe and steam you. Feel the joy of emotion.

Breathe in the warmth and allow it to fill you. When you feel any stresses in your body, let the gentle warmth of the sun relax your muscles and your muscles retain some tension.

When you imagine sitting there, if your mind begins to wander or gets engaged with daily problems (when thoughts appear to), just come back to feel the sun bathed you. Relax in the sunshine air.

This is everything there is to it! Just spend a couple of minutes in a safe place with a soft, golden light. There are no rules and you can change it for yourself. You can change the color from golden to any color you want. Perhaps you'd like to be bathed in purple or blue! Once you begin, you may wonder which color appeals most to you and go along with that.

You can create your own mini-holiday and experience the physiological, emotional and psychological benefits of meditation by going to your favorite place in mind and enjoying the sun's warmth.

Increasing your joy and feeling of well-being by giving yourself time. Give yourself a break from your constant occupation and allow your mind and body to relax. After a few minutes, you will feel more relaxed, renewed and back to your everyday life.

It pleases me to report that guided meditations are more and more popular with people who recently wanted to learn meditation. I'm particularly happy because I know how much they're doing.

The thing is, many people have difficulty meditating simply because nobody is there and can direct them through this process. Sure, directives like "Think of nothing" could be read. Yet I know that it's so much easier said than done, all too well.

Most people end up getting annoyed by meditations and end up leaving just because they're not entirely sure what they do. We don't see the outcomes everybody talks about, and we feel like they don't do it right.

It is no secret that it is easier for most people to be guided rather than teach themselves stuff, which is why I really like those meditations.

What is a guided meditation: a guided meditation is one that takes you through a trance. These can be in person, or you can listen to CDs and mp3s from your own comfort.

A soothing voice tells you exactly what to think about with this sort of meditation, encourages you to respire and helps you to stay focused. Once your mind starts to wander throughout the meditation, you will be filled with this soothing voice.

Guided meditations for all types of things are available. You can only get meditation to learn how to meditate or to learn specific things such as stress reduction, weight loss, relaxation, relationship enhancement, etc.

What this means to you: these meditations allow you to enjoy the benefits of meditation without having to become irritated and perhaps prematurely interrupt your practice.

CHAPTER 3

Benefits of Guided Meditation

A routine meditation practice is simply an outstanding way to cope with your stress. If you can relax profoundly in meditation, you feel much calmer, much calmer and less stressed when you are complete.

Stress can have many adverse effects on your body, particularly when it is felt for long periods. The relaxation experience restores you. It lets your body slip into a calmer place and provides deep rest and restoration. Such deep relaxation experiences slowly but surely reverses many of the damaging consequences of chronic stress levels.

Let's consider what this type of stress reduction technique is like. Guided meditation involves an instructor or a guide who directs and teaches you through the process of meditation and helps you discover relaxation, peace and perhaps inspiration.

He or she literally talks to you with soothing words, imagery and encouragement through this process. The words and ideas direct you to pursue your imagination.

The instruction is sometimes combined with peaceful music as well as natural sounds. You can actually allow the body to relax under the direction of the script as your consciousness focuses on the sounds of a voice or the music.

The benefits of this form of relaxation are many!

1. A guided meditation CD can provide you with the quality of meditation.

With a CD you can relax and unwind from meditation in the comfort of your own home, or wherever else you are because an audio product is convenient.

You have your own personal guide who can lead you skillfully to realms of deeper tranquility and peace. A guided meditation CD enables you to meditate and relax whenever you want. For today's fast-paced lifestyles it is the new way of wellness.

2. A guided meditation CD can make the meditation process easier for you and less effort.

Listening to the teacher's skillful instructions will enable you to remain focused through your meditation. A guided meditation CD can use soothing pictures of beauty, harmony and the world of nature.

Natural pictures may include the sights and sound of a quiet beach setting, the clear, light birdsong sound, the view of a peaceful lagoon or, perhaps, a noble mountain. These relaxing pictures encourage the mind to relax, and the body to relax, so that you can get a true sense of inner peace.

3. Guided meditation is user friendly.

Just lie back, turn it on, listen, follow the instructions. If you're a beginner, a CD is an effective way to relax. It is often the easiest way for you to experience the advantages of meditation quickly.

In fact, you will benefit from more meditation practice. It is helpful for those who find it difficult to focus and pay attention during a meditation experience. You are invited to engage your mind in the listening process with the audible direction provided.

This often allows you to remain focused so that your unconscious can more comfortably float into the calm, relaxed center, where you can enjoy the deep relaxation. You can take advantage of the therapeutic healing associated with meditation in deep relaxation.

We live fast-running lives today, full of demand, expectations and chronic stress levels. Excessive stress can have adverse effects on your health and well-being. Guided meditation is a useful and effective way to reduce the tension.

It is practical, user-friendly and available. Whenever you spend time relaxing with guided meditation, you can float into a place of significantly greater peace, deeper facility and health.

Using guided meditation is the easiest way for you to start meditation or continue regular meditation. Guided meditations are available in various formats, audio and video, and are meant to help you in a range of problems. In any matter ranging from reducing depression through to spiritual energy meditation, you will consider guided meditation.

The top three benefits of using guided meditations Better focus— people who have learned how to meditate and use guided meditation can remain focussed on the task at hand. You will relax completely and face a concentrated being the rest of your day.

Guided meditation goes through the emphasis on the topic of meditation, allowing the mind to concentrate on the purpose rather than the distractions normally present. By using guided meditation even five or ten minutes a day, the mind breaks away from all stress. This gives you a sense of calm.

Increase in Energy-You should be comfortable and even refreshed when your guided meditation has ended. You feel like you are ready to face the rest of the day and look past the root of pressure in order to find a good, consistent solution.

When you have reached the level of consciousness-led meditation, you can accomplish more and do what is required for others and for yourself.

In order to achieve this, you will need to train your mind from the normal, distracted one to the concentrated mind then to the meditating mind. It takes time to work through these three steps, but once you have learned it, it becomes easier and easier to get to the meditating mind.

Guided mediation is a great way to keep you up to date and reduce the negative aspects of stress. It takes just a few minutes and you will feel completely refreshed and restored.

If you have a large meeting that makes you nervous, take time for a little guided meditation and focus on the meeting. It can be used to recover calm in other ways, and it can only be a good thing in your life.

Great Reasons to Use Guided Meditation

1: You want to start meditating, but you don't know how!

Meditation brings healing to mind and body and opens up our hearts to love-and you can't really get much better. But if you have no meditation practice, it can be daunting, or even weird! Like walking with a trustworthy friend, you can go through this process through a guided meditation to learn how it works.

2: You've got ideas and triggers in your brain.

It's natural to distract thoughts-we all have them. But they can make it difficult to start the process of meditation. Guided meditation helps concentrate your thoughts on meaningful images to enhance the experience.

3: You've got a heart blocked.

Sometimes we are enveloped in the wrong things in the world we have seen. We're angry, not quiet, down to our core! Such thoughts will derail our meditation.

Guided meditation helps you to subtract the challenges of the moment, embrace love and go into the depths of your heart beyond the barriers.

4: You are afraid that when you meditate you will lift painful memories.

Most men with whom I worked with are afraid to meditate. "They know the dark spots in their lives, and in their hearts." How can I meditate when my heart is hurt so much? You know the pain, sorrow and grief deep inside. Moments of frozen rebellion, rays of helpless agony.

I was moved and inspired as guided meditation showed the very people that the sense of love and connection move through the risks, past the pain and deeply emotional comfort.

Therapy brings healing.

5: You want to share a friend's meditation.

A few years ago, one of my patients arrived at a pain management group that was thrilled after a week with friends on the lake. They strengthened their relationships and nurtured their hearts by guided meditation. They meditated together. It was an unforgettable experience.

Meditation is a profoundly moving practice and many people want to share it with someone they love. In reality, meditation can be even better when it is performed with others. A guided meditation enables you to easily introduce the process. Meditation can be shared with husbands, wives and even children.

6: For a while, you've been meditating, but feel a bit stuck.

Sometimes in our meditation journey we come to a dry place. Guided meditation shows a new way out of the deep paths that have left us stuck, and enables us to experience meditation in new ways.

We often find paths to areas we were never before! In the experience of the Source of All Love we have sought for all our lives, we can explore new aspects of love and mercies, forgiveness and grace, comfort and hope.

7: This is fun.

Meditation should be a serious business, I know. I know. And I guess that's it. Yet God is the wellspring of joy, happiness, and yes, fun! And when we meditate, we spend time on all good things with the Living Origin!

CHAPTER 4

What Makes Guided Meditation Different?

Many conventional meditation techniques allow you to monitor your own consciousness by focusing your attention on a single focus point. This concentration could be your breathing, it could be a physical action or more commonly a mantra-a tone, phrase or sentence you repeat mentally.

While these effective methods of meditation are great for inner quietness and increasing your focus, it is difficult for some people to master them.

One of the main reasons why guided meditation is so common as conventional meditation techniques is because it does not require previous training or effort.

Especially if you're someone who finds it incredibly difficult to leave thinking, even if you're highly stressed or overwhelmed with mental activity, your inner peace and mind is easily accomplished by being well directed.

Since this kind of meditation is so simple, it is very useful for new people. Nevertheless, guided meditations can also help people who are skilled in meditation.

Experienced meditators often use guided visualization meditations to undergo a deeper or more vivid meditation, deepen their minds as they usually are capable, or to concentrate on a particular aspect of their individual development.

Guided meditation also differs from conventional meditation by using music and sounds from nature to improve the meditation. The role of music and sound in guided imaging meditation Guided imaging meditation recordings typically include soothing meditation music that helps you relax during your meditation. Think of how much a good soundtrack makes for a film. Guided meditations benefit equally from music. Music brings to your guided meditation journey another layer of speech and complexity, thus relaxing your mind.

It is also not uncommon to include natural sounds for guided meditation CDs and MP3s. Such sounds are very calming and can also be used to boost the vibrancy of your visualizations during meditation.

For example, if you are directed to imagine yourself on a sandy beach, the visualization experience will be more realistic when you can actually hear the sound of the waves on the sea.

Contrary to conventional meditation, where mental stillness through relaxation exercises is achieved, guided imaging meditations rely upon a vibrant tapestry of visualization, music, and ambient sounds to calm, captivate, and immerse yourself in an inner journey.

Because this inner path can be adjusted for specific results, guided meditation may be even more effective when positive personal improvements are carried out in your life than conventional passive meditation techniques.

Guided Meditation-What are they and how are they working?

Guided meditation is, simply "guided" meditation. It is one of the simplest ways of achieving a state of deep relaxation and inner calm and one of the strongest ways to remove anxiety and make positive change.

How is it? How is it? How's that?

Guided meditation is usually done with a meditation teacher or a video.

A guide to meditation may ask you to sit comfortably, lie down. You are listening to your guide instead as you go through a series of calming views. As you relax gradually, anxiety fades away and your mind becomes clearer and clearer.

When your subconscious is in this very relaxed state of mind, it is open to constructive ideas and this time the Guide will take you on an inner journey to improve one or more aspects of your life.

For example, a guided meditation can be adapted to confidence and positive thinking. Another could focus on emotional or spiritual healing. You may take a guided journey to unlock your full potential, or a guided journey for deep relaxation.

As you can now see, guided meditation can be an experience not only of relaxation but also of self-confidence, transforming your dream into positive aspects and encouraging you to live life to the fullest degree possible.

It is a smooth and enjoyable experience that contributes to deep relaxation, stress relief and enhanced life enjoyment.

Your guide should slowly return to a normal state of awareness after your meditation, which will enable you to feel refreshed, rejuvenated and relaxed.

A guided meditation, depending on your preference, may take as little as five or an hour. In most cases, you are advised to take a 20-minute guided meditation if you want a truly deep relaxing state and reap positive benefits.

CHAPTER 5

Guided Meditations Help Transform Your Stress Into Calmness

There is simply no time to meet all requirements in one day. If we do not meet these demands, we feel stressed and pressured. Stress will impact our health in effect. You may want to consider practicing meditation because of our daily pace.

I may have lost you at this point as the next question is how do I find 10 to 15 more minutes a day through meditation? The mere thought produces another stressful series. To stop chatting, remember for a while that meditation can be done wherever and whenever. Yeah, you read it right.

If we can find the valuable minutes to spend, we can open ourselves to a calmer mind and to focus more on fulfilling the daily demands of our lives. The meditation practice helps us understand our own minds better.

Through investing 10 to 15 minutes a day, we will open up to tension managing, inner peace and happiness. Guided meditation can use the aid of a teacher or guide to turn our thinking processes from negative to positive, distressed to relaxed, and sad to satisfying through visualization.

To order to make our stressful life easier and more productive, the secret to guided meditation is to use as many senses as possible, such as tastes, sights, sounds and textures, to help create a visual image.

The goal is to achieve a deeper state of relaxation or consciousness than contemplation. The teacher or guide will easily imagine you to answer questions or problems.

The cognitive benefits of meditation include having a new insight into stressful situations, helping build stress management skills, growing self-awareness, reorienting / refocusing current ideas and reducing negative emotions.

Researches have shown that our health can be affected by stress. Stress can often be seen in allergies, anxiety, asthma, binge eating, cancer, depression, tiredness, heart disease, high blood pressure, pain, sleep problems and even violence.

Most healthy people use meditation to calm their bodies and reduce stress. Meditation helps facilitate physical and emotional well-being with any medical condition which may be aggravated by stress.

Throughout meditation, you focus your attention and remove the stream of "internal debate," which often overwhelms your mind and causes stress. You remove the overload of mind which grows every day and also contributes to our stress.

Visualizing photos helps you to see solutions to your problems, produces a balanced inner and outer being and focuses on positive results. The advantages do not end when the exercise stops, but can help you move more peacefully throughout the day.

The simple truth is that meditation is fast and cost-effective and requires no special equipment. The beauty is possible everywhere, at any time since we are in constant contact with one of our senses at any time.

How often do we wait for something or someone?

Did I activate one of your senses so you could meditate every day for these ten or fifteen minutes?

You have just begun (or ended) your day on the right note by listening to a guided meditation CD during your journey to work. Perhaps think about the time you spent waiting for your appointment in a doctor's office.

During this time, you can use this time productively for a major reason, and that is you. You should imagine the moment to calm your mind and body. The point is that you need not go to a yoga / meditation class to benefit from guided meditation.

Nevertheless, if you want assistance from a teacher or guide, you can find online resources for online support on different websites and using audio devices such as Dvds, etc. Try and do what works for you.

Stress Relief and Guided Meditation

You are tossed up, every day you are pulled out of your inner direction; this is what we call guided meditation. Stress relief and guided meditation is when you pay attention to these pushes (signs) and feel the urge to spend time. Feeling this guided meditation makes you feel stronger, because of course you contribute to inner calm.

If the nudges are gone, the nudges are constant until you really take care of them and do something about them. Taking this consistency into account can require not only meditation, but also exercise and eating the right foods. Many of the reasons why we feel stressed are due to our lifestyle.

Guidance comes inside...

There is a piece inside you that wait and want silence. This is an urge deep inside your sole that actively tries to remove the burden and alleviate you. The joys are what you want, and therefore your inner direction. The subconscious creates thoughts in your mind over and over and over again and tries to confuse you by manipulating you during meditation.

The subconscious is able to protect you from feelings of concern, anxiety and fear. Meditation is when the mind calms, the body relaxes, the muscles loosen, and the thoughts pass through you. Meditating 15 minutes or more a day will help relieve tension beyond language.

Only imagine encouragement and meditation will lead you somewhere else, like a wildflowers field or the beach. You then start to feel your being's softness and see how necessary it is to imagine your well-being.

You become one with the moment, and what you do in this imagination does not matter, because you let go of this reality. Even for a moment, leaving stressful life experiences can have lasting effects. Only imagine...

It is very important to pay attention to what happens after you meditate. Listening After Meditation You may not know right away what to do, but the questions you have previously had may no longer matter.

The worries and questions you previously had will have answers. Gradually as you get used to meditation, you will see that meditation is the most important part of your day and then signs.

Meditation life is the move to your truth. When you follow this path of stress relief and guided meditation and listen to the signs, you know where and when to sleep.

Meditation takes your life closer to the other side of your truth. It shows you the stairway to your life, and once you reach the top, every time you stay, every signpost, every path in bliss.

CHAPTER 6

Guided Meditations - Calm, Soothe, And Center

If you only have to pick one change in your everyday routine that would have a profound effect on every aspect of your daily life, you could choose practice or stop smoking. You can give up or detoxify caffeine.

It would be nice to do daily yoga. Nevertheless, the best choice is to devote an hour to guided meditations. No other exercise or wellness activity is physically, socially, mentally and spiritually more effective than guided meditation.

"Truly?" you ask. Who's got an hour to meditate? You know that you want to do it, but you don't know when, when or how. You point out, "I barely have time to floss and clean."

But who is so insane that an hour of meditation is not set aside? Apply a little logic to your busy, stressful and usually overcrowded life: wouldn't you find an hour to visit her if your sister is in the hospital? Why don't you spend an hour on your own health?

Do you not love yourself or care for yourself as much as you do for your sister? What if all your Facebook time was diverted to guided meditations? You will find that one hour of intense, calming and restorative meditation is more enjoyable and productive for the other 23 hours.

More than relaxing, controlled meditations combat tension.

We tend to underestimate our own mental power and also underestimate the strong, primordial link between our minds and our bodies. In a new romance, you "have butterflies" in your stomach when you still say the name of your lover if you can keep it mysterious and synchronize it with your heart beats.

When you think about the big meeting with all your colleagues and supervisors on Monday morning, your belly churns and your pulse turns into the red line. Psycho-physiologists believe that this link between our brains and survival is one of our oldest congenital patterns in the wild.

Nevertheless, we can monitor the relation between our thoughts and our biochemical reactions. Guided meditations allow you to suspend conscious thought and to break the link between the brain and the pancreas.

Once you pause your mind, the reflexes of fighting or flying are passive to avoid the release of stress chemicals. Your blood vessels are widening and taking the metabolic by-products of stress generated lactates out of your muscles. You should feel relaxed.

Guided therapy reduces pain as effectively as opiates.

The strain of the muscles exacerbates pain. The more you think of your pain, the more tense your muscles are and your pain increases. Opiates fill the dopamine receptors of your brain with fine chemicals, suspend your stress responses, make you feel good, and so ease your pain.

Powerfully addictive, opiates are physically even more addictive because it feels so good to feel so good, of course. But without the nasty side-effects, we can benefit from guided meditations. Our bodies secrete endorphins, many of them, as we meditate. Like opiates will, our natural sensational chemical products bind the dopamine receptors and we experience the same relaxation, satisfaction, and peace.

CHAPTER 7

Guided Meditation Can Help Fight Depression

Depression can sometimes prove fatal. People feel depressed for different reasons, and unless they are treated immediately, the illness may have an impact on their life indefinitely or at least permanently.

Depression affects the attitude and actions of an individual in ways that they never anticipate. It is therefore critical that you fight and treat depression the right way.

Although Saints and religious people are applying various methods to combat depression, certain approaches are not related to a particular religion, cast and race, but are available to everyone.

Meditation is a very helpful tool which should be used not only in times of distress but also every day. This direction will lead to happiness and personal growth. Although meditation helps you to feel good and to give a positive environment, it is also helpful if you are looking for emotional and mental relief.

There are numerous forms of meditation, Sahaja being one of them. Everyone can easily and quickly learn this method. This uses inner energy and boosts the mental and emotional health. Sahaja is not a new practice or a modern one. Yes, it is nearly a century old, and it is more common today, as its advantages have been scientifically proven.

The meditation of Sahaja began in the East somewhere. Their skills and strategies are universal, however, to allow people from all over the world to use them to fight depression. Sahaja promises a life-changing experience in a peaceful and happy future.

It lets you rid yourself of all negativity. It also promotes a healthy lifestyle and assures your well-being. Sahaja meditation not only allows you to overcome depression, but also helps you learn different ways to avoid depression.

There are many benefits of Sahaja and zero excuses not to pursue this guided technique of meditation. It also helps to increase your confidence and build trust, helping you to follow your dreams and goals without fear. It offers you an escape path so you can simply relate to yourself and to the world.

You should pay undivided attention to yourself and find ways to get out of various difficult situations. Sahaja's great thing is, you don't have to break the bank for it.

You don't have to spend an exorbitant amount of money on medications and can improve your life in ways that you might not have believed possible. Most websites offer guided meditations to Sahaja at no cost.

When you feel that you are emotionally depressed or have emotional difficulties, you should try Sahaja meditation as an alternative than to see a doctor or take medications. Many people from different parts of the world are finding peace and happiness by this approach with the same problems as yours.

This will help you to communicate with them, share and learn from your experiences. In this process, you will make new friends who have encountered and are able to connect with the same circumstances.

The biggest limitation we face when we do a guided meditation, or just meditate, is that our intelligence is getting in the way. We cannot stop thinking long enough to let the mediation system go and float. The root of this problem is terror.

What's the fear of meditation about? Typically it doesn't have much to do with the intellect. We are all afraid— an accumulation of anxiety which has been added to every time anything bad happens to us.

The more we've been wounded, physically or emotionally, the more we've got residual anxiety. (Unless we have, of course, done the internal work to relieve it. This is where counseling enters.)

Anxiety will begin to interfere with the way we live a normal life if we hold enough. Ultimately, it can be completely paralyzing. Yet luckily we have this operating device, called the ego, with us to help.

The ego gets a bad rap, but it's not a bad thing, really. His job is to help us stay upright, travel through life, and do stuff. When we have a lot of fear, the ego will try to help us not feel so much fear in order to do it. If we don't feel the fear, it won't slow us down as if we're always in contact with it. Good job, ego! Good job, ego!

One way the ego helps us not to be scared is by holding us in the head. They cannot be at the same time in two places so if we're thinking in our heads, they don't have any interaction with our heart where fear appears to occur.

Another way to say this is that the ego holds us in our mind to give us a sense of control.

When we are in our minds, we don't have more power over life, but the only thing we need is the sense of control, to keep us out of fear. The intelligence is like a safety blanket.

And we never want to let go of a safety blanket. This would make us awkward. And that's why the brain won't let go when we try to meditate. Unconsciously, anxiety keeps us trapped.

Guided meditation to deal with fear directly will be challenging, since you need anxiety out of the way to have an successful session. But if the anxiety is out of the way, you won't have to sit. It's complicated, but not impossible. It's not impossible.

CHAPTER 8

Reduce Stress With Guided Meditation

The rapidly moving lifestyle of today creates tension in all aspects of our lives. We are pressed to do more in shorter periods at work, at home and at leisure. Our physical and emotional wellbeing and well-being are affected by stress. The intense stress strain will age us faster and weaken the immune system to protect our immunity.

Most stress work environments record increased heart attack events at the workplace. You can do something once and for all to reduce stress. Guided or visualization meditations are a reliable and effective way to reduce stress.

While meditation is associated with monks who are seated in a mountain retreat, it is a proof method in order to combat stress and establish a healthy way of life for those of us who are involved in a fast-paced world. To beginners, guided meditation or visualization (two ways of explaining the same technique) is the place to start.

Guided and visualized meditations are soothing scenes in the background with calming music. The person on the CD instructs you to envision, imagine or talk about the less stressful situation that the guide shares with you. The photo is usually easy to connect with, such as walking in the woods or sitting on a remote beach.

Several scientific studies have confirmed that meditation is a successful way of treating stress conditions. Research studies have shown that meditation has helped to reduce blood pressure, lower diabetic blood sugar and lower levels of anxiety. Dr. Oz, who frequently appears on Oprah, recently suggested meditation as the first stress reduction process.

There are many advantages of meditation:

1. Increases levels of energy.
2. Clear perception of relaxation.
3. Concentration increased.
4. Reinforces the immune system.
5. Slows the process of aging.
6. Improves imagination.
7. The intuition awakens.
6. Helps reduce dependency.
9. This reduces stress. Heat.
10. Increases smartness.

The benefits of beginning a meditation practice extend beyond the 20 minutes you put into practice. If you relax deeply in a calm and peaceful environment, it offers a mini-vacation for your body. It's like you're peeling off tension and stress layers and discovering the true one outside this stress-filled combat environment.

Meditation sessions reset to normal and controlled your internal computer. In addition to the feeling of tranquility and relaxation, the brain fog becomes clearer and you are able to concentrate better.

Guided meditation provides deeper relaxation. You may not necessarily feel restful or energized while you sleep. When you meditate your entire mind and body, you relax. You're not sleeping. You are not involved in the sensations of the outside world. The methods you use instruct the body to relax and the body reacts.

All the listeners need is to turn off their phones and find a peaceful place to sit down and listen to the guided CD for 15-25 minutes. The commitment is low-buying a guided meditation CD and practicing once a day.

Choose a quiet spot when you begin your meditation practice and ask others who live with you to not disturb your meditation. Choose a time of day that's perfect to meditate on. Wear clothes that are loose and comfortable. Allow a few moments to sit down and reflect before you go back into your busy day. It allows the sense of deep relaxation to be incorporated into all aspects of your being.

You can still relieve or decrease your stress level instantly by guided meditation or use prescription medications that stress the body in a number of other ways. Meditation can be done anywhere, almost everywhere. Stop the persistent sense of confusion today! Meditate!

CHAPTER 9

Releasing Your Illusions - A Self-Guided Meditation to Help You Heal

On the surface, all delusions seem to be real. You wouldn't be fooled by them otherwise. If you look at them, you will find that the deeper truth does not help them. They are at the root wrong. Uncovering your delusions is one way of your soul growth.

Why would you first of all have believed in an illusion? You might have trusted in some delusions because they coincided with your own false beliefs.

But as you evolved spiritually, you started resonating with deeper truth and are less sensitive to lies and disappointment. Now you can easily feel the illusions. And thus you learn to recognize and remove from your heart and mind delusions and eliminate the false alignments of your lives.

In some situations, people may have deliberately deceived you. And sometimes, because of their own delusions, people confuse you accidentally. Yet remember this hidden truth before you rush to condemn one of them— Eventually, it is plain to you that you just fooled yourself.

This self-deception involves strength of character. You can slowly learn to listen to the deeper knowledge of your soul. And you also develop your ability, as you know, to use your common sense, intuition and thought. And through your observations, every day you become a little wiser. You can now move on.

You co-created this situation on some stage. You had to know something, and that was how your soul decided to learn. That is why you are ready to think about whether judging others or judging yourself. You know that this was the price of learning your lesson.

About this meditation: This self-oriented meditation is designed to help you understand yourself as a being that develops and learns. You must learn to release judgment energy, so that you can move on. You put the body, mind and soul together.

Allow yourself to use your imagination as you read each part of this meditation quietly. Take the time to feel every idea when you read it. Let the inspired feelings be incorporated into your being. Explore your consciousness ' spiritual healing powers.

Remember that you are cherished, because there is a deeper universal love that transcends your comprehension. Picture this universal love force, even though it doesn't seem evident at the moment...

Know that there is love and breathe it into your being, allow yourself to access your reality. You can now discover your deeper ability safely. This discovery has been waiting for your soul, so that you can live more authentically...

Breathe protection. Breathe safety.

You are more than your delusions, and you have greater potential than you know. Illusions should be known as false limitations. Realize the ability even if you can't yet sense it resides inside you. Your potential awaits you as an energy, and now you assert your potential–even though you're not sure exactly what it may be...

Consider and now breathe in the life of your higher potential.

Respire softly, thoroughly and attentively. Once you realize your breathing, you are now ready to live from a deeper, truer position. Note that your conscious breathing...

Take a breath into the deeper truth and see that you are becoming increasingly more secure.

You will move through moments of disappointment, self-judgment, disillusionment or frustration when you let yourself see an illusion for what it really is. That's ordinary. You don't dispute the decision. You must bless the power of judgment that exists to restore and release it...

You imagine the judgment— your own, or of anyone else — dissolving in the light of healing.

Now you feel your breathing. The breath grounds you in the reality of your divine existence, because you now feel everlasting spirit. Let fear or anxiety overflow. Look at it, let it go, layer by layer...

Let this recognition of your deeper reality emerge with every breath you take.

Let out of you the strength of the old delusions, like clouds of energy wafting softly. Let them slowly free themselves, disappear into small bubbles and note the subtle changes in you. If you release old energy of illusion, you remove deeper layers of illusion...

Don't judge old confusions when they emerge–just release them, like a mist that evaporates.

Recognize the more true and strong everlasting essence of yourself than the illusory patterns created. When you remove delusions, the knowledge of your everlasting spiritual inner reality increases...

Bless your inner light— your sacred reality— and be mindful that this is your true strength.

Think that you can go further than your delusions, because now you are going in a safer direction. When you feel your breathing at once and feel your reality, you take decisive steps on your journey of liberation and empowerment.

Imagine opening the better path in a healthy direction before you.

Now you look into the empty space where the illusion was in yourself. Maybe this room is now simpler and quieter. Perhaps even a little clean. That's all right. But what are you going to do with this space...

Bless where the illusion was in the empty space.

You put your favorite truth where the illusion was in that old space. Perhaps you want a new image to be put there. And new thoughts and new ideas. Or maybe you're not sure. That's all right. Only bless it, ask for love, comfort, empowerment, or whatever is right...

Respire the energy of the new healthy picture, and let your new energy flow easily.

Bless yourself, bless your body, bless your mind, bless those concerned and bless the universe...

Let everyone be cured, in its own unique way, as you thank all and everything.

You know that all facets of that condition are also supported by the universe. And you've been given the ultimate blessings...

Respire with every breath in the eternal divine blessings that cure every part of this situation.

You continue to breathe, breathe with air, and moment by moment, as you become one with the love and grace of the Godhead. It increases the vibration so that divine grace, divine reality, divine love, and divine wisdom can be obtained.

Allow yourself to breathe the strength of God's grace softly.

Well done, thank you now for leading yourself through this soothing meditation. All happens for a reason and you addressed your delusions with confidence and are now preparing yourselves for divine grace to pour into your life.

When required, you can perform this self-guided meditation and will be amazed each time you experience it to discover new empowerment opportunities within you. As you read the words to yourself, slow down, take a moment to remember your breath and visualize each step of the meditation.

You are going forward, the world blesses you, and you choose a positive path. May single step forward inspire you in marvelous ways.

CHAPTER 10

Guided Meditation Using Binaural Beats

The use of binaural beats is a relatively recent development of the practice of meditation. Binaural beats had both objective and subjective effects on consciousness states.

The technique is used to create varying, stable states of consciousness by manipulating those brain wave frequencies. This enhances individuals ' ability to experience a profound state of meditation where the brain adapts to new perspectives and achieves propitious, changed states of consciousness that create a wide range of beneficial effects.

Binaural beats are produced by two coherent signals, which are delivered one to each ear at slightly different frequencies. The brain understands the phase variations between the sounds and listens to a binaural rhythm.

Normally, it provides spatial information to the person when a phase difference in sounds is detected. That is, from that direction comes the sound. Nevertheless, the brain absorbs all sounds and detects a third sound, the binaural rhythm, when this phased difference is viewed by stereo headphones.

During binaural beats for guided meditation, the typical frequency of the brainwaves is less than 30 Hz. Hearing these beats at various frequencies induces unique awareness shifts that are directly linked to the frequency used. Beats between 1 and 4 Hz that suit the delta state usually reproduce high amplitude brainwaves that are typical of slow wave sleep.

The frequencies tend to make him fall asleep when the person is tired. With a frequency of 4 to 8 Hz corresponding to theta brainwave levels, subjects regularly report a calm, dreamlike trance and deep relaxation, frequently marked by imaginative sparks.

If the binaural rhythm varies from 8 to 12 Hz, the effect on the alpha frequency, which is the frequency of wakeful sleep, or the dreaming with closed eyes, is more pronounced.

It is considered the ideal level for enhancing cognitive processes, such as learning and memory, because of increased concentration and alertness. It is the fact that athletes sometimes find themselves "in the field."

But how does guided meditation help with this technology?

The best way to prepare your brainwave training ability effectively is to lie on a comfortable bed in a quiet, peaceful space. The darker and quieter the better, since the goal is to reduce external sensory input to a minimum, so that the brain can travel inside without disrupting the senses. The use of an eye mask can be effective as well.

Another approach, especially in experimental environments, is the use of a sealed flotation tank in which the subject is suspended in a boiling, skin-like liquid in an enclosed sensory environment.

The subject begins the mp3 meditation until relaxed and immerses itself into the sound of the headphones.

The binaural beat produces in the awake, varying and repetitive effects depending on the chosen frequency and the accompaniment of the associated "pink" sounds, which consist of music, natural sounds and a changed white hiss such as the television, when the channel is tuned to avoid transmitting.

These include: relaxation, improved creativity, insight, in-depth meditation, enriched learning, enhanced sleeping habits, well-being and personal discovery of altered states of consciousness.

Such effects start quickly and automatically using binaural beats. The subject must not try to achieve deep meditation. The beats training process creates a profound alteration of consciousness that can be used to draw upon the incredible imagination and capacity of the human brain to solve problems. G-meditation with binaural beats concentrates on a specific frequency to induce a known desired effect.

Guided meditations can be used to improve abilities, including, but not limited to: sp, imagination, vivid visions, memory, perceptions, happiness, anxiety reduction and spa.

The use of binaural beats in guided meditation will shorten years of effort to achieve a deep state of meditation. One thing is sure, these beats are going to change your mind

CHAPTER 11

Guided Meditation Mp3s - How To Quickly And Easily Achieve Total Relaxation And Peace Of Mind

In this segment, I will introduce you to guided meditation MP3s, a fun and powerful method to achieve meditative relaxation and peace of mind quickly and easily.

Meditation has been used in many cultures around the world for thousands of years to help people relax and live healthier lives.

There are various forms of meditation. In some cases, the aim is to create a transcendental experience. In other aspects it is targeted at having a deep understanding and addressing personal problems. The object of the most basic forms of meditation is simply to relax and experience peace of mind.

One difficulty with meditation is that it can be hard to get it right. While meditation on the surface is simple, requiring nothing more than sitting still and relaxing the mind, the committed practitioners may spend years or even life perfecting their meditation techniques to achieve the desired results.

Most people meditate with the best of intentions, only after a short while to give up dissatisfaction. Sitting still and quieting the mind can be a very difficult task in today's busy modern world. Guided meditation MP3s offer a way to obtain the same outcomes as advanced meditation, but in some situations.

Binaural beats are one of the most common forms of guided meditation MP3s. Binaural beats are the result of the left and right ear (such as in a pair of headphones) receiving two slightly different auditory waves separately to enable neurophysiology to create a similar, consistent pattern of brain waves that generates a high level of relaxation and sensitivité.

Meditative, binaural beats are achieved with the simple MP3 audio of relaxing music or naturally occurring sounds with the two sounds which activate the binaural beats which have been inserted in the music.

You only have to sit or lie down comfortably, close your eyes and listen to the fun audio path through your headphones to enjoy their meditative effect. Only beginners are not rare to feel a deep sense of relaxation and peace of mind just five or ten minutes after listening to a album.

Among the many common benefits of listening to binaural beats are better sleep, increased consciousness and imagination, increased energy, deep relaxation, better meditation, lucid dreaming and even out - of-body experiences.

CHAPTER 12

Yoga Guided Meditation Options To Begin

Most people find that doing yoga a few days a week helps them to stay in shape and to increase flexibility over time.

If you want a routine that will help you relax, meditation is the ideal tool for relaxation. You can do this at your own speed and in your own home's privacy. When you want to do this, beginning with yoga-guided meditation is a good idea.

Yet finding the right one can be a bit daunting, because there are essentially several choices available. The key to finding the right guided session is to take a while to weigh your options, rather than choosing your first one.

There are many sources out there, so how do you know which one for you is perfect? All depends on your level of comfort and how much money you are willing to spend. Be mindful that some solutions are more expensive than others.

It is also worth remembering the old adage, "You get what you pay for," which often occurs in guided meditations. Others prefer those who focus primarily on meditation, while others prefer different types that require various stretches and offer body toning after each session.

A very successful meditation guided yoga alternative is to hire a personal skilled trainer who can teach you and motivate you to take the different yoga poses. A qualified trainer will customize a session that meets your needs exactly.

He will also devote his time solely to showing you how to execute every yoga pose correctly so that you can make the most of every session. Sadly, this alternative is also very costly.

The majority of professional trainers bill the hour. When you decide to take this option, you will want to make sure that during each session you get right to business.

If you are a gym or fitness center already in your city, see if there are any qualified trainers in your gym who perform guided yoga meditation lessons. Most sports facilities now include free classes for their participants.

You can still learn the basic yoga poses and how to do them properly while you cannot get a personalized session in this way. Once the yoga poses of these classes are mastered, you can do them at home every time you have time.

When you are not a gym or are not really happy with a yoga class, a yoga-guided meditation option for you is a yoga meditation DVD. Many such DVDs are available online and offline today.

Such DVDs will help you learn the best privacy strategies at home and at home. You can adjust the techniques in yoga-guided meditation DVDs to make them easier and more enjoyable for you and to suit your specific needs.

CHAPTER 13

Techniques for Guided Meditation

There are different strategies or methods to make it speechless or track the constant noise stream that it likes to generate. Most times, the mind appears to be a force all for itself, an adversary residing in one's own body.

But let us not forget that the true purpose of the mind is to serve the true self, its master. The mind is a device to achieve several things. The mind can even be used as a meditation course. Guided meditation is one of the many relaxation forms. At the end of a Yoga class, guided meditations are often held.

The power of human imagination is immense and this mighty force makes directed meditation so successful. The individual envisages predefined scenarios and these photographs produce a profoundly meditative state.

The recommended visualizations must be either recalled from the memory or heard through a speaker, or a video, since the eyes are closed; reading is not a choice.

One can record and listen to the recording in advance or they can ask a friend to repeat it for them as some people interrupt the sound of their voices during guided meditation. Any approach that works best for a person is their best path.

The unconscious mind cannot distinguish fact or fiction; everything with which it is presented is accepted as fact. That's why we fear a scary film or we cry at the end of a tearjerker. The conscious mind understands that a film is not real, but it is true to the unconscious mind. It happened to that level of the mind. With our imaginations, the same can be said. The stuff we dream of in the realms of the imagination also affect our processes physiologically. When we are concerned, the heart rate rises, the palms become sweated, and the breath grows shallow, quick, or both.

Normally, this important part of the mind is unconsciously and never consciously used, which is great potential waste. The unconscious mind becomes a great tool for deep internal change with guided meditation.

Comfort should be considered before joining the guided meditation. Wear loose fitting clothes and position the body comfortably over the long distance. Settle down in the chosen position and wait one or two minutes. If further changes are required, do so now. The meditation can start once the body is taken care of.

There are multiple guided meditations to choose from and each has its own advantages. Pure light meditation means that the light is clearly perceived and absorbed in the body; it is purifying and purifying as all the impurities and psychological wounds contained inside it are removed.

The notion of becoming one with a tree, down to the bark rawness and the feeling of soil around the tree roots, is another example of guided meditation. This is a basic meditation.

There are countless guided meditation examples to choose from, each of which has different effects. The trick is to choose what you are attracted to as an individual based on your specific needs.

CHAPTER 14

Guided Meditation Script - The Best Way To Achieve A Deep Meditative State

The fastest and easiest way to achieve a deep meditation is through a guided meditation script and guided meditation audio CD. They are also helpful for advanced yoga novices.

There are meditation audios that use isochronic tones or binaural beats which have an impact on some areas of the brain at explicit frequencies.

These audio CDs are available in any shop containing yoga DVD products and other Yoga resources. You can also easily find these products online.

How do Scripts of Meditation Aid Meditation?

In essence, a teacher can read a guided meditation script in a Yoga class during Savasana to bring the class into a deeper level of relaxation.

An example of this is a Yoga Nidra meditation text. Some audio CDs have tonal stimuli with Isochronic, Binaural and Monaural beats that guide practitioners to better meditation. We examine these in detail below.

1. Monaural beats

Monaural beats are stimuli imposed on one pulse and continuously filled in other soothing sounds at a single pitch. It's more like a warm afternoon's soft liquid sound of a sluggish ceiling fan.

The vibration produces a hypnotic effect and the calming can be heard. You can even start to doze off. Monaural beats act in a similar manner but produce substantially different results.

2. Binaural beats

They are repeated beats that are segmented to each ear at different frequencies. When the difference is between 10 and 30 Hertz, the brain makes the difference by producing another sound that compensates the difference.

Thus the conscious mind gradually begins to harmonize with the pulse of the tones. Binaural beats are designed to quench the conscious mind and clear the clutter of thoughts and pave the way for the subconscious mind to articulate its creativity.

3. Compared to the above, Isochronic tones are produced by spacing the tone pulsations equally at much higher frequencies which leads to a greater pace of synchronization of the brain with the pulses.

The soothing sounds of the sea, the water and the wind are superimposed on music and create an effect of the constant bubbling away of our minds.

It has been found that isochronic tones are much more effective than monaural and binaural beats when used in guided meditation. Isochronic tones help practitioners reach a relaxed mood and a deep meditative state very quickly.

4. Guided Meditation Script

The more passive the practitioner is, the better results will be. A guided meditation script requires very little effort. You simply need to relax and listen to the soothing sounds of rain, wind and music on CDs or yoga DVDs, or read someone from a guided meditation writing while surrendering, de-stressing and taking advantage of them.

CHAPTER 15

What To Do With A Guided Meditation Script?

If you think you can't do much with a guided meditation file, think again. A list of things you can do here, and this is only the tip of the iceberg.

At the end of the day, relax.

Concentrate your mind for the day.

Recover your strength and rebuild it.

Touch and restore the past.

Chart your future goals and your path through life.

Brainstorm thoughts by removing visual filters.

Sharpen your intuition. Shape your intuition.

Overcome fear. Overcome fear.

Become a more affectionate person.

Disable mental disorder.

Get some true, old-fashioned time for silence.

Return to the Almighty.

Research subjects by engaging individually with them.

Branch out with new insight in new directions.

Bring unwelcome character traits to the surface and resolve them.

It's just the tip of the iceberg, as I said. Your guided meditation script is restricted to your imagination only.

One thing I want to say is that you don't go crazy with many different meditations. It appears to interrupt the post. One or two a day, ideally in the morning and/or in the night.

If you are writing a whole bunch of different meditations and then running through all of them on the same day, it probably won't be as good as doing only one or two guides a day.

One good thing about your own script is that you can customize your images. You can do a guided meditation that leads to an occurrence and then a new meditation that allows you to solve it.

As you can see, meditation does not have to be somewhat frustrating, annoying, because you have to chore. You can use a guided meditation script to improve every aspect of your life, if you find or write good ones.

Over time, you may find that the meditation practice fuses into your life activity. The benefits of meditation are not limited to certain times, and meditative thinking is not confined to practiced meditation. Instead, you will gain access to your tools at will and find that your mind is sharper and harder to counteract harmony.

As with any ability, day-by-day progress is difficult to see, but you start with a guided meditation script and have a month or two review with yourself in the future to see how you perform. I think you're going to be pleasantly surprised.

CHAPTER 16

Set The Scene To Give Your Guided Meditation Script A Boost

When you are planning to use this guided meditation template, you can use a few things to give it a real edge. It has to be a couple of minutes more can make a big difference in quality.

Let's just step back and remember that the goal is to get the participant (or meditator) to concentrate on the meditation, not anything. Not only do you avoid distractions by providing a good setting, you can also boost and enhance the efficacy of your guided meditation script.

Let's begin with music. When dealing with meditation alone, I find that with soft music in the background it tends to work easier. I have a few rules I use when I pick such music: it must be free of lyrics (instrumental or sometimes words without voices). It can't be too quiet or too vibrant. It ought to be soft and gentle.

Ultimately, it must be as unstructured as possible. Think of music as a gentle path that never seems to go, but has a nice scenery. That's the music we want for your guided meditation script as history.

You can pick music with properties that complement the meditation if you want to be imaginative. For instance, you might include music using ocean waves if you have a meditation that uses beach pictures. Instead, if you are in the mountains or the forest, it is best to record forest sounds (unless it is obtrusive / busy).

Also, we try to make our environment as calming and safe as possible, so that you can truly work with your guided meditation script. Make sure the room isn't too hot or cold, and you might want to put a smell in the air.

There are many ways to add a scent in the breeze. You can go for the desired effect with sprays, candles, heated essential oil, incense or any variation of the above container. I also have a few suggestions for the sound background: make sure it is friendly and accessible.

Those of us who are used to incense can tolerate more exotic scents, but you want to concentrate not only on watering eyes and coughing but also on what is in your guided meditation guide. Don't overdo it on the same page. A little is a long way away.

Remove artificial fragrances. It can be less expensive, but often the smell only gets dressed rather than comfortable. Once, we want to focus our attention on the inside.

Compare the form of scent with the individual. If they do (and some people do) respond to incense, instead use candles or heat some essential oils.

Once you put all these together, the meditator is almost immediately comfortable and your directed script is so much more successful. There is a bit of an art here, so continue to test and see what works best for you.

How To Make a Guided Meditation Script Work For You

Whether you intend to use guided meditations or guided images, make your own guided meditation script. While it's easy to go and hear a guided media recording, I'd like to ask you: Have you ever listened to such a recording and come up with the idea that it wasn't written for you? In this chapter, I will teach you how to adapt existing meditation scripts to your needs and how to document them for yourself.

Nothing needs to be said for having a professional connection while listening to a guided meditation, but I find it much more beneficial to listen to guided imagery that is explicitly suited to your needs. Only try to act like you're a kid calming. Keep it clear, keep your voice quiet. Don't add scary videos unless you intend to deal with them.

One of the easiest ways to get started is to take and rewrite an existing directed picture script. Easy enough, it has three very good purposes: to show you how the script is written and how it flows. It can give ideas on how to make your own originals, not least–it helps you to adapt the script to your own mind (or for another-family member, relative, etc).

In any case, once you have a personalized guided meditation file, you may want to turn it out. When I come up with new directed images, I do. Apparently, guided meditation does not work too well if you read it (although this too can be mastered by practice).

You have two options: option one is for somebody to read to you, and that is an annoyance to you both. If you want it to be flawless before you show that, it can be a bit embarrassing. The second option is to record it and play it back to yourself. Obviously, I am in favor of option two.

It is simpler than you could imagine to record your guided meditation script. (Not so many) Years ago a tape recorder would have done this. It was rather linear and very difficult to edit. It's very easy to record on your computer nowadays.

There are two great free apps that I use and recommend: Audacity and CD Burner XP Pro. Audacity is a completely free audio recording program and CD Burner XP Pro is a free CD burning program based on Windows.

You can record and edit your directed image session with these two programming (with audacity) and then record to CD if you don't have a CD Burner XP Pro (MP3 player). D the combination of these two programs together with the already available information means you can use an existing guided meditation template, tailor it to your needs, and then have it at your fingertips whenever you want.

Better still, you can share it with your loved ones. Over time, you may find that you have created the entire directed picture library tailor-made for yourself and your loved ones.

You know nothing beats experience, so start with a small guided imaging session and see what happens when you customize it for you. The results could surprise you.

CHAPTER 17

Guided Meditation - Achieving Complete Control And Concentration

In essence, the art of meditation not only allows us to discover profound inner peace and relaxation, it also allows us to grow as people.

But some people get the wrong feeling that meditative relaxation simply is a waste of time, a hippy event, or only for people with serious mental problems. We don't understand the practice of meditation to sharpen one's mind and give a positive direction and a new perspective in life.

Similar to other practices, meditation with a true sense of purpose should be performed. For example, when you apply for a new job, you are intentionally, right? When hired you receive a salary that you spend on clothes, food, holidays, living expenses and general fun. People do not usually work if they do not have such a goal.

Meditation is similar. You must have a meditation purpose that may differ in its methods.

Meditation practitioners do so to gain inner tranquility, discover new levels of concentration, improve your general presence of the mind, open up new learning opportunities and promote creativity, work towards self-healing, take control and responsibility for fears, address sleeping problems, etc.

One general aim in meditation cannot be provided because each person has their own individual goals and challenges to overcome in life.

It's easy to just release tension and bring your relaxation to a new level with guided meditation because there is always someone there with you to make sure you do it right to your goals. It is therefore extremely important that you carefully select your meditation guide.

Every meditation specialist and practitioner follows a different kind of strategy. We make it easier for people to explore the many forms of meditation according to their goals.

The majority of meditation instructors start with deeper breathing techniques that lead you to relaxation and concentration. Meditation techniques certainly won't work if you can't focus on breathing. Note, each guide is different from another guide. So ask the meditation professional for a free meditation session before you participate in ongoing sessions.

Even in one single meditation group, teachers often have their own style and way of bringing you into a relaxed state. Make sure you go to someone who really knows what you are trying to do. You may wish to challenge yourself, for example, with fresh meditation ideas and ideas for which you can purchase one of the performance guided meditation CDs.

You're trying to settle for it, but after a few minutes, you break into laughter peals. The voice sounds completely unreal because it is perfected electronically. So this method will not help you to get everywhere you need to focus and relax, while the same CD will sound normal and function for someone else perfectly.

Take your selection from other versions of meditation. The local bookstore or Internet will help you find direct audio and video tracks for meditation. But don't run and buy anything you see, go to the samples first if they are available. Remember to think about accents; a meditative cd with a British emphasis may not be appropriate if you are from the USA.

Fine quality meditation snippets are generally open for viewing and testing. This is quite similar to booking a meditation center or health spa for yourself. Eventually, guided meditations can only work if you are disciplined enough to practice your lessons regularly.

CHAPTER 18

How To Use Guided Meditations To Awaken And Utilize The Power Of Your Mind!

If you are able to take the first steps towards a better life, you have to find someone to walk through the fundamentals of meditation. Those who heard guided meditation CDs have experienced increases in creative problem solving, improved concentration, and reduced stress and tension.

Guided meditation takes you through easy to understand and apply exercises to strengthen visualization. These exercises help to strengthen the connection between your body and mind to improve mental focus and acuity. You deserve a better life and meditation will lead to peace of mind and stress-freeness.

I have been teaching meditation since 1981 and have developed a line of meditations using relaxation methods to address everything from stress management and insomnia to weight loss and abundance. If you're a person who doesn't accept the' body-mind' energy, how can you explain what's going on with your body when you engage in sexual fantasy?

The mind is so strong and so powerful in our lives that we fail to use it for our own good. Many people fear and think about the future they consider what could go "wrong" instead of what could go "true."

You have no time to register for a 3-day relaxation program if you are like most people. Guided meditation is the ideal way to achieve a busy way of life. The discovery of audio recordings to help you, step by step, learn how to meditate, is like getting your own personal meditation instructor at your side, 24 hours a day, 7 days a week.

No more books for reading, just press the play and close your eyes and you'll meditate like a master in minutes. It was never simpler and some tips on finding a good guided meditation are given.

1. Is background music there? Music relaxes your brain's right (creative) part, while the led voice relaxes your brain's left part (analytical). Aim to use a guided meditation with ambient music to help the whole brain relax.

2. Does the leading voice calm you and sooth? Make sure you pick a guided meditation that you like to listen to with a male or female voice.

3. Find a place you won't be bothered. Turn off your phone, close the door and let your family know that for 30 to 45 minutes, when listening to the guided meditation, you don't want to be interrupted.

Make sure you sit down or lay down on a couch in a favorite chair. Don't sit in your bed to meditate. Your subconscious mind connects your bed to sleep, and during your meditation you may fall asleep.

4. Wear comfortable loose clothes.

5. So help you relax faster, apply lubricating eye drops to each eye until meditation is closed. This can easily calm and relax your face. Relaxed eyes allow the entire body to release stress faster.

6. Practice listening to 2-3 separate meditation titles to practice various techniques for relaxation.

7. Let your mind soar. Let your mind soar. Be as imaginative and creative as you can when the words are spoken, let your entire body, mind and spirit really concentrate and hear the words. Learning the fundamentals of guided meditation opens your mind to experiences you never thought.

CHAPTER 19

Guided Meditation And Regression - Powerful Tools For Transformation

Guided imagery meditation and regression are modes used more frequently in the past couple of years and are effective instruments for transformation and empowerment.

What is guided meditation in imagery? Therefore, directed meditation is a combination between relaxation, hypnosis, and meditation in which a deeper stage of consciousness is triggered and a position somewhere between the waking and the inconscious or sleeping state is achieved.

We can go "back" and quiet outside forces and disturbances in this state to reach our inner core. Different types of images may be used depending on what the guided meditation attempts to do.

Since visualization is being used, this modality draws on our imagination and may make it easier for us to pull "onto" the meditation and to break barriers which could otherwise have hindered answers.

Guided visualization therapy for a variety of purposes may be used. It can be used for calming, tension and relaxed anxiety. It can be used to get feedback and spiritual guides to touch our Higher Self. It can be used to face and tackle fears and resolve them.

It can be used to cope with and treat childhood issues. It can be used to gain self-esteem and love of oneself. And as we try to move actively through life, it helps us to plumb our own depths, to better understand ourselves, and to bring unconscious things to consciousness.

One of the very positive aspects of guided meditation with pictures is that it helps us to find our own answers. It is therefore a strong motivational device. The professional using this technology will assist his or her customer's empowerment mechanism rather than simply giving the customer information that he / she could have sought or telling the customer what to do.

For the customer it can be a powerful and transformational experience to follow its own guides and find their answers and can significantly accelerate its own healing, development, and empowerment cycle. Spontaneous changes and emotional breakthroughs can occur.

In addition, a professional and intuitive practitioner can tailor the session to your needs and can really also "be there" and feel how the photos and therefore the experience are guided.

This can yield much better results than can be obtained by programmed guided meditation tapes that may not be specifically tailored to your needs (although tapes can certainly be beneficial instead of individualized sessions).

Regression sessions are similar to directed visualization therapy, where a calm state is triggered and a person's consciousness is brought to a deeper level. Regression of age or past life can be accomplished either through directed imagery or through a more simple approach.

The key component of regression sessions is to be taken to another time–usually at a younger age in the present or past life.

For various reasons one can regress: dig into childhood issues and the underlying causes of pain and fear, in order to make understanding and breakthroughs easier; investigate past lives to identify possible triggers of life problems, worries, relationships, etc., past lives; etc. Regression can also be a powerful tool for change and help to create ideas and breakthroughs.

One can also go into the future in one's lifetime, or into the future. This technique can be called progression.

When best, guided meditation on imagery and regression / progression can be powerful tools for self-transformation and empowerment with a non-invasiveand facilitative benefit. The uninvasive and simple approach to these approaches allows you to go your own way, find your own answers and motivate yourself.

CHAPTER 20

Choosing A Guided Meditation

About anybody can record a guided meditation. That's fine, except you're looking for a good person to use, so there's a lot to do. Here are several things to look for when you choose a guided meditation to ring your bells (softly, of course).

Samples.

There is no reason to buy a web audio recording without hearing a sample at this stage. And you'd rather consider a seller to send you a generous sample of a minute or more, so what you get is a good idea.

If the sample is 30 seconds or less, you will wonder what they are trying to hide. Of example, the author is limited to the website's 30 second requirement if you are looking at websites such as Amazon or iTunes. But those rules do not apply on the publisher's website.

Talk. Voice.

It is important to be comfortable with the voice of the narrator. How do you feel when you hear? Will their voice sound attract you and make you comfortable? Does it concern you, or do you just want to nod?

There's a trend for guided meditation, hypnosis, and leading visualization voice artists in a monotonous way, because some artists think that's the way to get you into a deep transformation. Ultimately, this is the way you lose interest.

No excuse the speaker can't add a dramatic aspect to your reading, almost as if they told you a bedtime story. The softness of the delivery is the strength of your voice, which allows you to deepen. The narrator should sound like they are interested and involved in what they say, otherwise why are you supposed to be?

Art history. Music background.

As with the sound of the narrator's voice, you can enjoy the sound and feel drawn into the background music. It ought not to sound "weird" or hokey, dry, friendly and welcoming. Unfortunately, as sythesizers became affordable, the world opened to millions of artists who wanted new ages and music quality went down quickly on the market.

Holding a chord on a soft pad for 20 minutes is not an effective way to create a backdrop of music. A good music backdrop for a guided meditation would suit the theme of the script emotionally. It should preferably be explicitly written for the software.

Text. Script.

The story and the letter will draw you in and make your journey relaxed, safe and welcoming. Again, writing a meditation is simple, but it takes some imagination and commitment to compose and rewrite until the script is a sophisticated work of art, making people want to listen over and over.

CPSIA information can be obtained
at www.ICGtesting.com
Printed in the USA
BVHW041748040321
601714BV00008B/526